Meriam Khadhar
Raja Trabelsi
Hanene Gaied

Prevention of infection in peritoneal dialysis

Meriam Khadhar
Raja Trabelsi
Hanene Gaied

Prevention of infection in peritoneal dialysis

What's real and what's not?

ScienciaScripts

Imprint

Any brand names and product names mentioned in this book are subject to trademark, brand or patent protection and are trademarks or registered trademarks of their respective holders. The use of brand names, product names, common names, trade names, product descriptions etc. even without a particular marking in this work is in no way to be construed to mean that such names may be regarded as unrestricted in respect of trademark and brand protection legislation and could thus be used by anyone.

Cover image: www.ingimage.com

This book is a translation from the original published under ISBN 978-620-3-44936-5.

Publisher:
Sciencia Scripts
is a trademark of
Dodo Books Indian Ocean Ltd. and OmniScriptum S.R.L publishing group

120 High Road, East Finchley, London, N2 9ED, United Kingdom
Str. Armeneasca 28/1, office 1, Chisinau MD-2012, Republic of Moldova, Europe
Printed at: see last page
ISBN: 978-620-5-66546-6

CHAPTER I

Peritoneal dialysis (PD) is one of the methods of extrarenal purification in patients with end-stage renal disease and receiving replacement therapy.In 2015, estimates suggest that 272,000 people are on peritoneal dialysis worldwide about 11% of the dialysis population [1]

PD is an ambulatory technique, but patients must be taught and educated beforehand by specialized nurses to minimize the risk of bacterial contamination during the maneuvers for connecting the catheter to the dialysate bags.Infectious complications are the most feared complications of this technique. There are two main types of infections: infections of the catheter outlet and infections of the dialysis fluid (peritonitis).These peritonitises occur essentially as a result of contamination during handling, or either by continuity following an infection of an orifice or in connection with a bacterial translocation through the digestive wall. The germs most frequently found are staphylococci, but gram-negative bacillus peritonitis is increasingly being diagnosed.In Tunisia, unfortunately, there are no national data concerning the incidence of peritonitis in PD. However, in

France, according to the French language peritoneal dialysis registry (RDPLF), the incidence of peritonitis is one episode every 32 patient months (i.e. 0.37 episodes per year) [2]. Although there are international recommendations for diagnosis, prevention and treatment from the International Society of Peritoneal Dialysis (ISPD) [3], the incidence of infectious complications remains high and variable from one country to another.Prevention in its various forms remains the central core of care.We found no articles in the literature interested in assessing young nephrologists' knowledge of preventive measures in PD.The objective of this work is to evaluate the theoretical knowledge and practical conduct of young Tunisian nephrologists in terms of prevention of infectious complications in order to detect the difficulties encountered and to remedy them, and then to take stock of the preventive measures of peritoneal infections in peritoneal dialysis.

CHAPTER II

I. Topics:

This is a prospective observational cross-sectional descriptive study that took place between June and July 2022 targeting young nephrologists. These physicians are required to complete an anonymous questionnaire distributed online. A total of 65 questionnaires were sent to the different physicians (residents in training and university hospital assistants). Forty-four physicians responded to the questionnaire (67.69%).

1. Inclusion criteria:

Young Nephrologists, residents and university hospital assistants.

2. Non-inclusion criteria:

Nephrologists who were not in practice at the time the study was conducted.Nephrologists practicing abroad. Associate professors and professors.

3. Exclusion Criteria:

There are no exclusion criteria since the online platform receiving the responses only accepts fully completed questionnaires.

II. Methods:

1. The questionnaire (Appendix):

The questionnaire consisted of 11 questions. Four on the status of the physician and the training he or she has had in peritoneal dialysis. Seven questions about infection prevention in peritoneal dialysis; 10 single choice questions and one multiple choice question.

The questionnaire was oriented towards the following topics:

a. Antibiotic prophylaxis and infections

b. Technical gestures and infections

c. Screening for and eradication of nasal carriage of staphylococcus aureus

d. Timing of the first dressing

e. Systematic local antibiotic therapy and infections

2. Procedures:

Questions 1 through 4 were descriptive in relation to characteristics related to the survey population.The remaining questions (7 questions) on the theoretical and practical knowledge of young nephrologists (residents and AHU) on infection prevention in peritoneal dialysis were scored out of 7. Each question was scored as either correct or incorrect. There was no possibility of a partial answer. The score was between 0 and 7.

The scoring of the responses was as follows:

• 0 : False answer

• 1 : Correct answer

The questionnaire was distributed by email and using social networks to young nephrologists. Responses were collected on the google form interface and by email for analysis.

3. Statistical analysis:

Data were entered using Excel and analyzed using SPSS version 23.0 For the descriptive study, we calculated simple frequencies and relative frequencies (percentages) for categorical variables. We calculated means, medians, and standard deviations and determined extreme values for quantitative variables.

Ethical considerations:

Anonymity was maintained throughout the study. No information on the identity of the participants was requested.

CHAPTER III

1. General Statistics:

Table I includes the mean, median, minimum, maximum and standard deviation of the questionnaire responses. Forty-four questionnaires were completed and validated. The maximum score was seven out of seven. The minimum score was one out of 7. Four physicians scored seven.

Table I: General statistics of questionnaire responses.

Statistics	
Average	4 45
Median	4
Standard deviation	1 5
Minimum	1
Maximum	7

2. Characteristics related to the study population:

1. Question 1: Are you a resident?

Thirty-four physicians who responded to the questionnaire were residents (77.27%). Six are first year residents (17.65%); Fourteen are second year (41.18%); Ten are third year (29.41%); Four are fourth year (11.76%). (Figure 1)

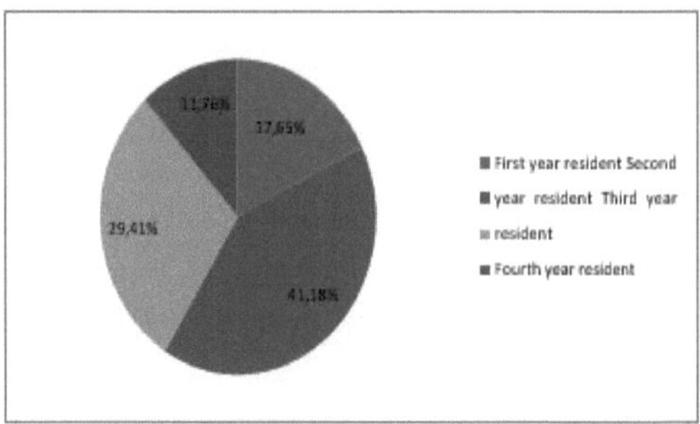

Figure 1: Distribution of responding physicians by year of residency.

2. Question 2: Are you a university hospital assistant?

Ten physicians (22.73%) are university hospital assistants (UHA). Two are first year AHU (20%). Three are second year UFAs (30%). Three are third year UFAs (30%). And 2 UFAs in the fourth year (20%) (Figure 2).

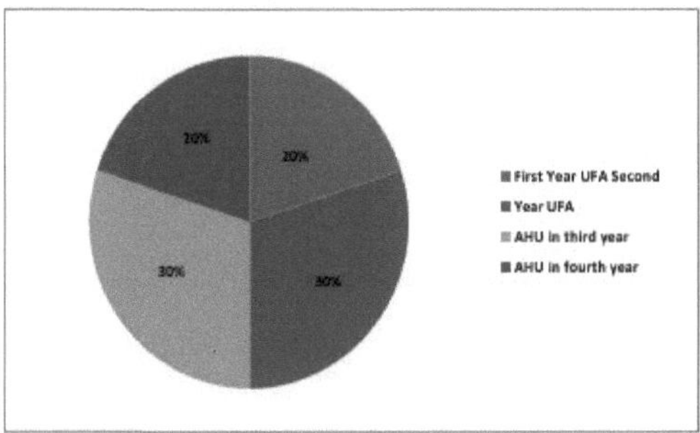

Figure 2: Distribution of physicians responding to the questionnaire by year of assistantship

3. Question 3: Have you had extensive training in peritoneal dialysis

To this question, 50% answered that they had not had any in-depth training. One physician had two advanced trainings (inter-university diploma in peritoneal dialysis and Baxter training in PD (Figure 3).

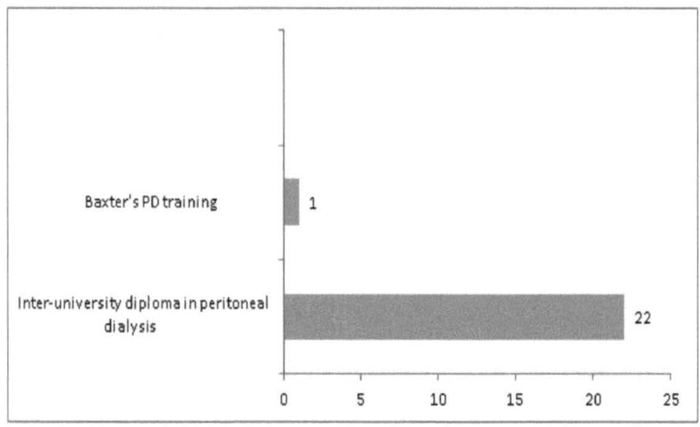

Figure 3: Distribution of responses regarding in-depth training.

4. Question 4: Did you go to PD during your exercise?

40.9% responded that they had not had a peritoneal dialysis placement for a minimum of 3 months (Figure 4).

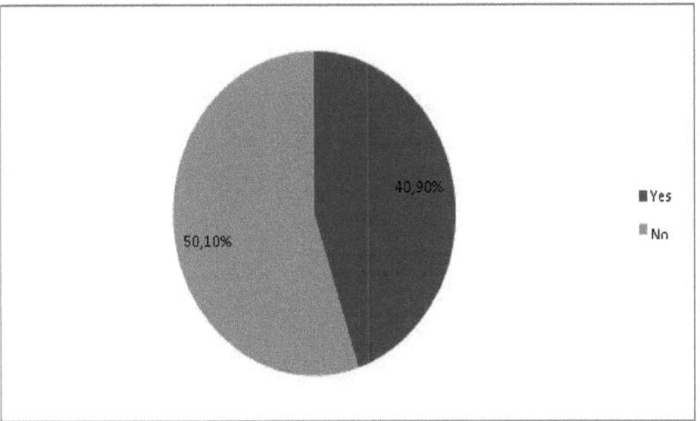

Figure 4: Distribution of physicians according to whether or not they had a peritoneal dialysis unit visit.

3. **Descriptive study of questions on theoretical and practical knowledge of infection prevention in peritoneal dialysis:**

1. **Question 5: In your opinion, does the use of a buried catheter (Moncrief method) reduce the incidence of port infections?**

More than half of the physicians incorrectly answered yes to this question, stating that protecting the catheter under the skin until it was necessary to initiate renal replacement therapy reduced the incidence of port infections. (Figure 5).

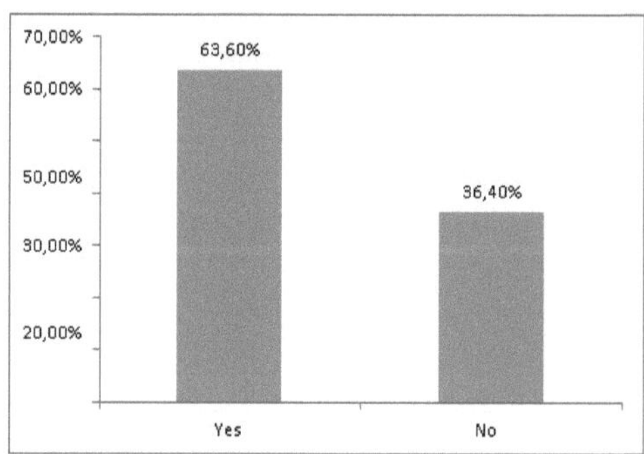

Figure 5: Distribution of responses regarding Moncrief's method and its impact on outlet infections.

2. Question 6: In your opinion, is an antibiotic injection in the preoperative phase recommended to decrease the risk of infection?

90.9% (n=40) of participants answered the question correctly. (Figure 6).

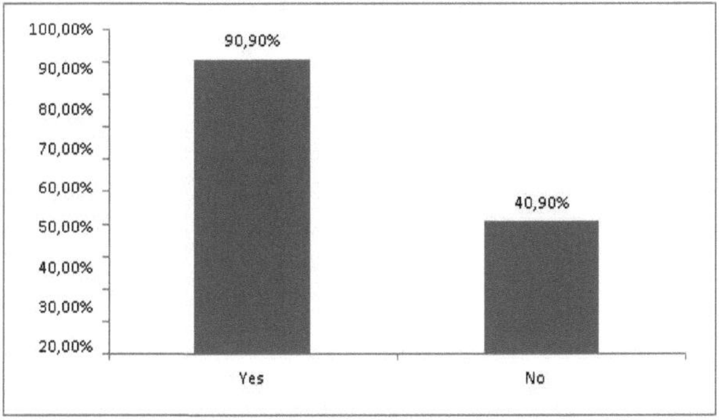

Figure 6: Distribution of responses regarding antibiotic prophylaxis

3. Question 7: In your opinion, should screening for nasal carriage of staphylococcus aureus be performed routinely after catheter placement?

Responses were mixed. 59.1% responded that screening for nasal carriage of staphylococcus aureus should be done routinely (Figure 7).

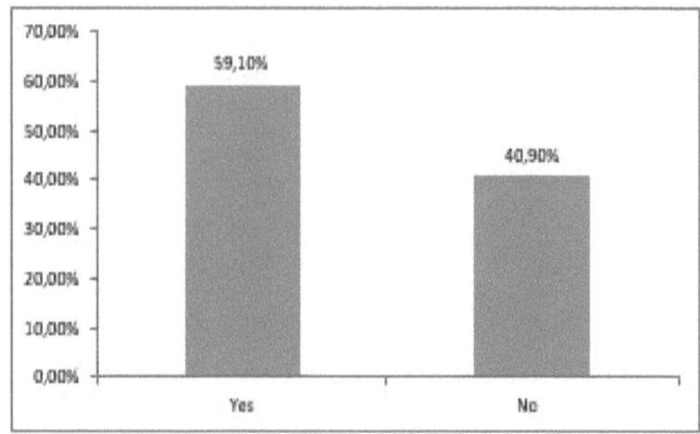

Figure 7: Distribution of responses regarding nasal carriage screening.

4 **Question 8: In your opinion, should eradication of nasal carriage of staphylococcus aureus be performed routinely in a patient undergoing peritoneal dialysis?**

Responses were also mixed. Just over half of the participants (n=24) answered no to this question (54.5%). (Figure 8)

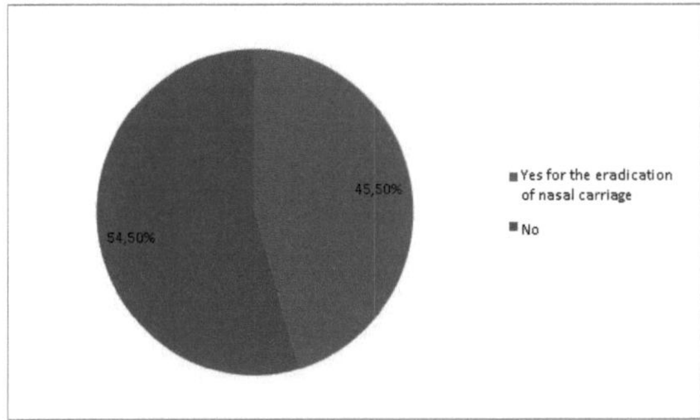

Figure 8: Distribution of young nephrologists' responses regarding eradication of nasal carriage in PD.

5. Question 9: In your opinion, intermittent systemic treatment is the best solution to eradicate nasal carriage

The majority of physicians (n=71) had a correct answer to this question. (Figure 9)

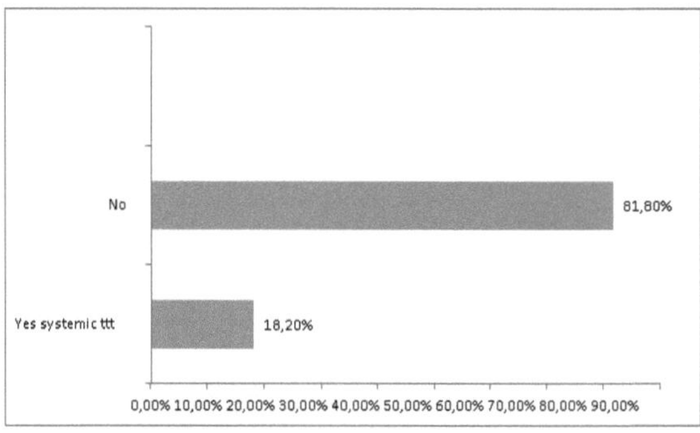

Figure 9: Distribution of responses regarding the means of eradicating nasal carriage

6 Question 10: In your opinion, is it common practice to do the first dressing seven days after catheter placement to avoid mobilizing the cuff and promote healing?

According to 68.2% of the doctors questioned (n=30), the first dressing should be reapplied within an average of 7 days after application (Figure 10).

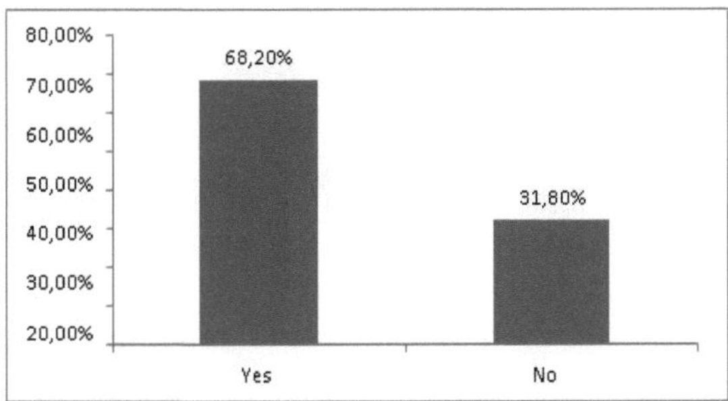

Figure 10: Distribution of physician responses by timing of first dressing.

7. Question 11: Do you prescribe a local antibiotic after the disinfection procedure to reduce the risk of infection?

To this question, 72.7% answered that adding a local antibiotic decreased the infectious risk (Figure 11).

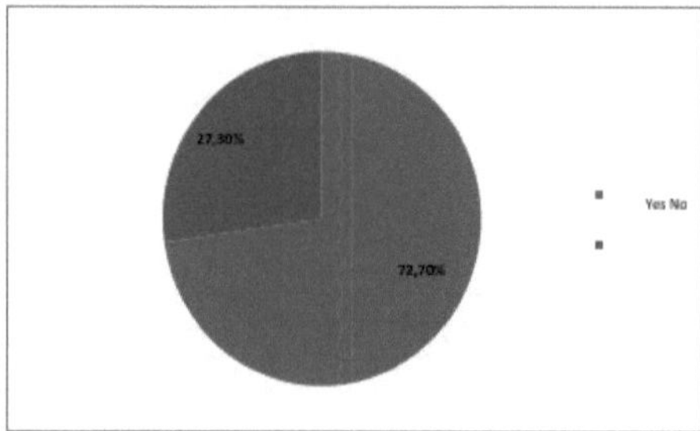

Figure 11: Distribution of physicians' responses regarding eradication of exit site carriage.

CHAPTER IV

1. Preoperative intravenous antibiotic prophylaxis:

An injection of antibiotics in the preoperative phase is recommended to reduce the risk of infection, especially early peritoneal infections. Gadallah et al [4] conducted a clinical trial including 221 peritoneal dialysis patients. Eighty patients received cefazolin, 86 patients received vancomycin and the others did not receive intraoperative antibiotic prophylaxis and they demonstrated that antibiotic prophylaxis significantly reduced the rate of peritoneal infection but not outlet infections.

Moreover, the latest recommendations published in 2021 by the Indian Society of Peritoneal Dialysis recommend the administration of a systemic prophylactic antibiotic before catheter insertion [5].

The ISPD also recommends intravenous antibiotics before insertion of a PD catheter [3]. This recommendation is based on 4 randomized controlled trials comparing perioperative IV antibiotics to no antibiotics[6].

This antibiotic prophylaxis must be of short duration, not exceeding 24 hours. Antibiotic prophylaxis should be adapted to the ecology of each center. Antibiotic coverage should include the Enterobacteriaceae family, as well as Gram-positive organisms commonly found on the skin flora. Indeed, the majority of organisms cultured from catheter port specimens are Gram-positive organisms commonly found on the skin, such as Staphylococcus aureus, coagulase-negative Staphylococcus spp. and Streptococcus spp. [7,8,9].

We of current practice in the hospital mongi slim la Marsa we prescribe 1 gram of vancomycin throughout the operative act of setting up the catheter of peritoneal dialysis.

90.9% of the participants answered correctly to the question: yes, antibiotic prophylaxis is necessary before the placement of a peritoneal dialysis catheter.

2. Moncrief's method : (buried catheter)

In 1991, Moncrief and Popovich introduced a new technique for PD catheter implantation. This catheter has a coiled tip with 2 cuffs and an arcuate bend between the cuffs. This would prevent leakage of PD fluid. Then they embed the outer segment of the catheter into the subcutaneous tunnel during insertion. The catheter segment is kept buried for 4 to 6 weeks before externalization. This procedure will allow time for tissue growth in the outer surfaces of the 2 sleeves, preventing bacterial colonization of the catheter surfaces from the exit port and thus reducing peri-catheter infections[10] .

The placement of a buried catheter (the so-called Moncrief method) is not one of the recommendations for preventing exit wound infections or peritonitis [3,5].

Indeed, opinions are divided. Several clinical studies confirm that this new catheter implantation technique increases catheter life expectancy and reduces peri-catheter infections. This was reported in the review of the literature directed by Dasgupta MK in 2002, 10 years after the invention of the moncrief catheter[11].

On the other hand, Osako et al [12] reported an infection of the exit orifice and the tunnel within 2 weeks of catheter exteriorization after the Moncrief-Popovich technique in 3.3%. The catheter malfunctioned in 1.9% after the Moncrief-Popovich technique due to occlusion of the catheter by a fibrin plug [12]. The ISPD concludes that there is no convincing data indicating that the buried catheter technique reduces the rate of peritonitis[13].

In our current practice, this technique is not used to prevent the risk of infection. More than half of the physicians answered this question with an erroneous yes, stating that protecting the catheter under the skin until it was necessary to initiate renal replacement therapy reduced the incidence of port infections.

Time to initiate PD after catheter placement:

Once the PD catheter is inserted, there is debate about the optimal time to initiate PD.The Timely study showed that there were higher rates of peritoneal fluid leakage when PD was initiated 1 week after catheter insertion compared with waiting 2 to 3 weeks [14-15].

Leblanc et al showed in 2001 that leaks are associated with outlet infections and peritonitis [16].

In our current practice, a delay of 3 weeks is observed before the use of the PD catheter. If the patient requires extra renal purification within 3 weeks, intermittent hemodialysis is used. The same is true for the first dressing, and it has been noted in current practice that delaying the change to 7 days mobilized the catheter less, gave less leakage and therefore less peritonitis. But there are no recommendations on this subject. The young nephrologists answered with a yes that a delay of 7 days should be respected in 68.2%. As there are no recommendations in this sense, this answer can be tolerated.

Nasal carriage of staphylococcus aureus (Screening-eradication-treatment) :

It is not necessary to carry out systematic screening for nasal carriage of staphylococcus aureus after catheter placement. Moreover, this common practice in the various peritoneal dialysis units does not constitute a recommendation of learned societies [3-5]. Indeed, carriage is frequent but intermittent. A negative sample does not exclude the diagnosis.On the other hand, it is not recommended to eradicate nasal carriage of staphylococcus aureus in a systematic way in patients undergoing peritoneal dialysis. Indeed, the "mupirocin group" working group had concluded, after screening 1144 PD patients in 9 European centers and subsequently randomizing 267 staphylococcus aureus carriers into two groups, that nasal mupirocin did not reduce the incidence of tunelitis or peritonitis. The ISPD just suggests screening for nasal S. aureus carriage before insertion of the DP catheter (Grade 2D)[17] . If nasal S. aureus carriage is found, they suggest treatment with nasal application of mupirocin (1B)[17] . This reduces the risk of infection of the exit orifice, but has no impact on the risk of peritonitis.In our current practice, we continue to take a nasal swab and if it is positive for staphylococcus we prescribe Oflomed 5 drops per day for 5 days every month. As a result, the responses of young Tunisian nephrologists were divided between recommendations and current practices.

Outlet care (eradication-treatment):

In the study of Amato et al. they demonstrate the same genotypic identity of the staphylococcus aureus found in the outlet and in the peritonitis [18].

It is therefore necessary to eradicate portage from the catheter exit port to prevent tunnelitis and peritonitis[5] .

With respect to treatment, rifampin 600 mg po daily for 5 days every 3 months reduces the incidence of catheter but does not reduce the incidence of peritonitis and is also associated with a high incidence of adverse events [19].

A meta-analysis showed that routine application of mupirocin to the port after the disinfection procedure reduced overall S. aureus infection rates by 72% and S. aureus peritonitis by 40%.[20]

Local mupirocin has equivalent efficacy to systemic rifampicin treatment but with fewer adverse effects [21].

In recent years, resistance to mupirocin has been reported, but it is more common with intermittent use than with daily use. [22-23].

Piraino et al found an increase in pseudomonas infections as a consequence of the extensive use of mupirocin ointment [24].

A comparison of gentamycin cream and mupirocin shows that gentamycin also reduces the incidence of infections [25].

The ISPD recommends daily topical application of mupirocin or gentamicin to the catheter exit site (grade 1B) [13].

The application of Mupirocin to the catheter outlet reduces the incidence of peritoneal staphylococcus aureus infections and the application of Gentamicin reduces the incidence of gram-negative bacilli and staphylococcus aureus infections and is therefore a good alternative to Muporicin cream [5].

In Tunisia, mupirocin cream is not available, but gentamycin cream is available, but given the risk of bacterial resistance to this antibiotic, it is not used. In current practice, the exit orifice is disinfected with betadine but no local antibiotics are applied.

Enhanced education reduces the incidence of infections

Education of the patient and health care professionals is essential. The duration and frequency of education sessions vary greatly. However, it is estimated that a minimum of 3 education sessions per patient is necessary. Both the ISPD and the Indian Society recommend that training be provided by nurses with appropriate qualifications and experience (Grade 1C) [3-5].

During the education process special attention must be paid to the learning of connections.After an episode of peritoneal infection, the need for further education of the patient and/or health professionals should be assessed.The "flush before fill" method should be performed systematically as it reduces the incidence of peritoneal infections (grade 1A) [13].

In Tunisia, there is an emphasis on patient education by experienced nurses, but there are no videotapes or brochures dedicated to this learning process to facilitate adherence to the educational program.

CONCLUSIONS

Peritonitis is one of the most dreaded complications in peritoneal dialysis. They can be a source of failure of the technique and death of the patients.The incidence of peritonitis in Tunisia is unfortunately not known as there is no national registry.Nevertheless, the prevention of infections in peritoneal dialysis relies on certain measures that the ISPD has detailed in several of its recommendations (guidelines) and updates: 2016-2017-2022.The objective of this work was to evaluate the theoretical knowledge and practical conduct of young Tunisian nephrologists in terms of prevention of infectious complications in order to detect the difficulties encountered and to remedy them, and then to take stock of the preventive measures of peritoneal infections in peritoneal dialysis.We conducted a prospective observational cross-sectional descriptive study between June and July 2022 using an anonymous online questionnaire. The target population was young nephrologists practicing in Tunisia at the time of the survey. Each physician had to fill in a direct questionnaire, oriented on the knowledge concerning preventive measures in peritoneal dialysis. The questionnaire consisted of 11 questions concerning the screening of nasal carriage of staphylococcus aureus and its eradication, antibiotic prophylaxis, surgical techniques, timing of the first dressing and local antibiotic therapy at the exit port. The data were collected and analyzed using SPSS 23.0 software. Forty-four physicians responded to the questionnaire (67.69%). The average score was 4.45 out of 7. 63.60% of the physicians answered incorrectly with a yes that protecting the catheter under the skin until it was necessary to initiate renal replacement therapy reduced the incidence of port infections. 90.9% (n=40) of the participants answered that yes, an antibiotic injection in the preoperative phase is recommended to reduce the risk of infection. Concerning nasal screening and staphylococcal eradication the answers were divided. 59.1% answered that screening for nasal carriage of staphylococcus aureus should be done systematically. For eradication, 45.5% answered that Eradication of nasal carriage of staphylococcus aureus should be performed routinely in a patient undergoing peritoneal dialysis. No intermittent systemic treatment to eradicate nasal carriage in 81.80% of responses. According to

68.2% of the doctors questioned, the first dressing should be reapplied at a distance from the application and this within an average of 7 days. Finally, 72.7% answered that adding a local antibiotic reduced the infectious risk. Our results show the confusion of some of our young Tunisian nephrologists and this is due to the fact that the practices of the service are not necessarily consistent with the recommendations of the ISPD. Some erroneous attitudes still exist among a good number of physicians; in particular that of screening and eradicating nasal carriage to reduce the risk of peritonitis in patients undergoing peritoneal dialysis.

Perspectives:

The incidence of peritonitis in PD patients remains high and variable from one country to another. In Tunisia, there is a project to set up a national dialysis register.

Given this confusion among young nephrologists between the ISPD recommendations and current practices in hemodialysis units, we must develop our own national recommendations and follow them. Moreover, a working group of the Tunisian Society of Nephrology, Dialysis and Transplantation is in the process of finalizing Tunisian protocols for the management of PD patients. Training courses dedicated to preventive measures in PD targeting young nephrologists and PD nurses will give them the opportunity to better master this technique. Practical training workshops on mannequins will allow a more concrete approach for those who do not have access to PD units during their training.

REFERENCES

[1] Fresenius Medical Care. Fresenius Medical Care 2015 Annual Report: ESRD patients in 2015: A global perspective (FMC 2015).

[2] www.bdd.rdplf.orgVolume 1, n 1, June 2018. https://doi.org/10.25796/bdd.v1i1.30; ISSN 2607-9917

[3] Philip Kam-Tao Li, Kai Ming Chow, Yeoungjee Cho, Stanley Fan, Ana E Figueiredo, Tess Harris , et al. ISPD peritonitis guideline recommendations: 2022 update on prevention and treatment. Perit Dial Int 2022 Mar;42(2):110-153.

[4] Gadallah MF, Ramdeen G, Mignone J, Patel D, Mitchell L, Tatro S. Role of preoperative antibiotic prophylaxis in preventing postoperative peritonitis in newly placed peritoneal dialysis catheters. Am J Kidney Dis. 2000;36:1014-9

[5] Tarun k Jeloka. Continuous Ambulatory Peritoneal Dialysis Peritonitis Guidelines - Consensus Statement of Peritoneal Dialysis Society of India - 2020. Indian J Nephrol. Sep-Oct 2021;31(5):425-434

[6] Strippoli GF, Tong A, Johnson D, Schena FP, Craig JC.

Antimicrobial agents to prevent peritonitis in peritoneal dialysis:

a systematic review of randomized controlled trials. Am J

Kidney Dis. 2004;44((4)):591-603.

[7] Scalamogna A, Castelnovo C, De Vecchi A, Ponticelli C.

Exit-site and tunnel infections in continuous ambulatory

peritoneal dialysis patients. Am J Kidney Dis.

1991;18((6)):6747.

[8] Nessim SJ, Komenda P, Rigatto C, Verrelli M, Sood MM.

Frequency and microbiology of peritonitis and exit-site infection

among obese peritoneal dialysis patients. Perit Dial Int.

2013;33((2)):167-74.

[9] Hildebrand A, Komenda P, Miller L, Rigatto C, Verrelli M,

Sood AR, et al. Peritonitis and exit site infections in First

Nations patients on peritoneal dialysis. Clin J Am Soc Nephrol.

2010;5((11)):1988-95.

[10] Moncrief JW, Popovich RP, Broadrick LJ, He ZZ, Simmons

EE, Tate RA. The Moncrief-Popovich catheter. A new peritoneal

access technique for patients on peritoneal dialysis. ASAIO J.

1993 Jan-Mar;39(1):62-5.

[11] Dasgupta MK. Moncrief-Popovich catheter and

implantation technique: the AV fistula of peritoneal dialysis. Adv

Ren Replace Ther. 2002 Apr;9(2):116-24

[12] Osako K, Sakurada T, Koitabashi K, Sueki S, Shibagaki Y. Early Postoperative Complications of Peritoneal Dialysis Catheter Surgery Conducted by Nephrologists: A Single-Center Experience Over an Eight-Year Period. Adv Perit Dial. 2017 Jan;33(2017):26-30].

[13]Li PK, Szeto CC, Piraino B, de Arteaga J, Fan S, Figueiredo AE, et al. ISPD Peritonitis Recommendations: 2016 Update on Prevention and Treatment. Perit Dial Int. 2016 Sep 10;36(5):481-508.

[14] Ranganathan D, John GT, Yeoh E, Williams N, O'Loughlin B, Han T, et al. A randomized controlled trial to determine the appropriate time to initiate peritoneal dialysis after catheter insertion (Timely PD Study) Perit Dial Int. 2017;37((4)):420- 8.

[15] Leon Hsueh, Susie L. Hu, Ankur D. Shah. Periprocedural Peritonitis Prophylaxis: A Summary of the Microbiology and the Role of Systemic Antimicrobials. Kidney Dis 2021;7:90-99

[16] Leblanc M, Ouimet D, Pichette V. Dialysate leaks in peritoneal dialysis. Semin Dial. 2001;14((1)):50-4.

[17] C Szeto, PK Li, DW. Johnson, J Dong, AE Figueiredo. ISPD catheter-related infection recommendations: 2017

UPDATE. Peritoneal Dialysis International, Vol. 37, pp. 141-154

[18] D Amato 1, de Jesus Ventura M, G Miranda, B Leanos, G Alcantara, M E Hurtado, R Paniagua. Staphylococcal peritonitis in continuous ambulatory peritoneal dialysis: colonization with identical strains at exit site, nose, and hands. Am J Kidney Dis. 2001 Jan;37(1):43-48

[19] SW Zimmerman, Perit Dial Int 1991; 18:225-231

[20] Xu G, Tu W, Xu C. Mupirocin for preventing exit-site infection and perito-nitis in patients undergoing peritoneal dialysis. Nephrol Dial Transplant. 2010;25:587-92.

[21] Judith Bernardini BSN Beth Piraino MD Jean Holley MD James R.Johnston MD Ronald Lutes DO. Am J Kidney Dis. Vol 27, No 5 (May), 1996: pp 695-700

[22] Lobbedeez T, Gardam M, Dedier H, Burdzy D, Chu M, Izatt S, et al. Routine use of mupirocin at the peritoneal catheter exit site and mupirocin resis-tance: Still low after 7 years. Nephrol Dial Transplant. 2004;19:3140-3.

[23] Al-Hwiesh AK, Abdul-Rahman IS, Al-Muhanna FA, Al-Sulaiman MH, Al-Jondebi MS, Divino-Filho JC. Prevention of peritoneal dialysis cath-eter infections in Saudi peritoneal dialysis patients: The emergence of high-level mupirocin

resistance. Int J Artif Organs. 2013;36:473-83.

[24] Piraino B, Bernardini J, Florio T, Fried L. Staphylococcus aureus prophylaxis and trends in gram negative infections in peritoneal dialysis patients. Perit Dial Int. 2003;23:456-9.

[25] J Bernardini J Am Soc Nephrol 2005; 16:539-545

APPENDIX

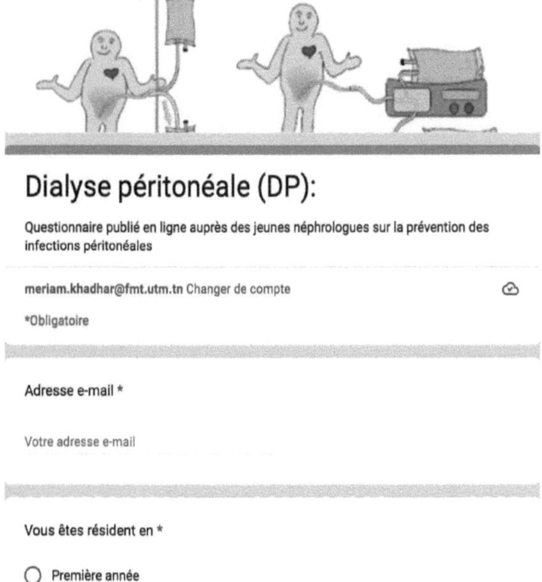

Dialyse péritonéale (DP):

Questionnaire publié en ligne auprès des jeunes néphrologues sur la prévention des infections péritonéales

meriam.khadhar@fmt.utm.tn Changer de compte

*Obligatoire

Adresse e-mail *

Votre adresse e-mail

Vous êtes résident en *

○ Première année

○ Deuxieme année

○ Troisieme année

○ Quatrième année

○ AHU

Vous êtes AHU en *

○ Premiere année

○ Deuxieme année

○ Troisieme année

○ Quatrième année

○ Résident

Es ce que vous avez eu une formation approfondie en DP *

☐ Non

☐ PD forum Baxter

☐ Diu en DP

Es ce que vous êtes passé en DP (minimum 3 mois) lors de votre exercice *

○ Oui

○ Non

La mise en place d'un cathéter enfoui (méthode dite de Moncrief) réduit *1 point
l'incidence des infections d'orifice

○ Oui

○ Non

Une injection d'antibiotique dans la phase préopératoire est recommandée *1 point
pour diminuer le risque d'infection ?

○ Oui

○ Non

Un dépistage du portage nasal de staphylocoque aureus doit être réalisé de *1 point
façon systématique après la pose du cathéter ?

○ Oui

○ Non

Une éradication du portage nasal de staphylocoque aureus doit être *1 point
réalisée de façon systématique chez un patient en dialyse péritonéale ?

○ Oui

○ Non

Un traitement systémique intermittent est la meilleure solution pour éradiquer le portage nasal * 1 point

- ◯ Oui
- ◯ Non

Ajouter un antibiotique local après la procédure de désinfection permet de diminuer le risque d'infection ? * 1 point

- ◯ Oui
- ◯ Non

Il est de pratique courante de faire le premier pansement 7 jours après la pose du cathéter pour ne pas mobiliser le cuff et favoriser la cicatrisation * 1 point

- ◯ Oui
- ◯ Non

Envoyer

Effacer le formulaire

Ce formulaire a été créé dans Université de Tunis El Manar. Signaler un cas d'utilisation abusive

Google Forms

TABLE OF CONTENTS

41

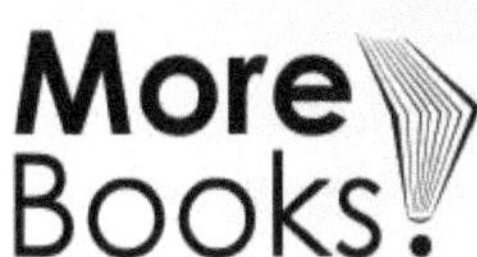

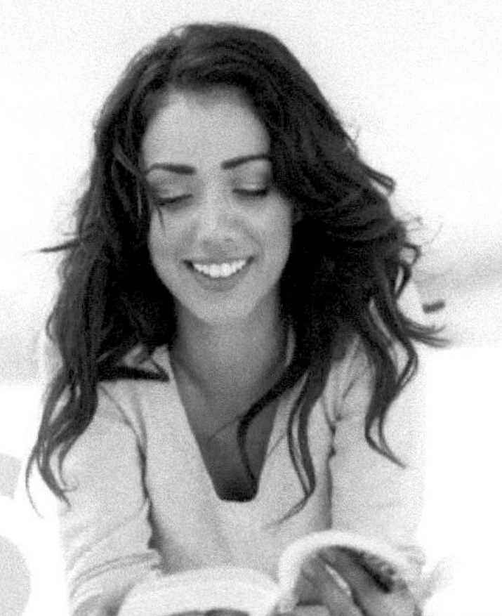

yes
I want morebooks!

Buy your books fast and straightforward online - at one of world's fastest growing online book stores! Environmentally sound due to Print-on-Demand technologies.

Buy your books online at
www.morebooks.shop

Kaufen Sie Ihre Bücher schnell und unkompliziert online – auf einer der am schnellsten wachsenden Buchhandelsplattformen weltweit! Dank Print-On-Demand umwelt- und ressourcenschonend produziert.

Bücher schneller online kaufen
www.morebooks.shop

info@omniscriptum.com
www.omniscriptum.com

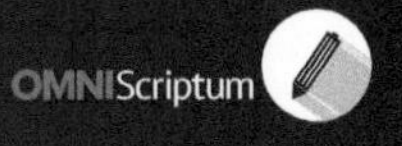

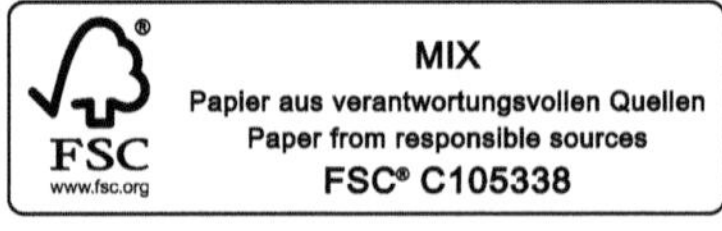

Printed by Books on Demand GmbH, Norderstedt / Germany